Heart Disease and Aortic Aneurysms

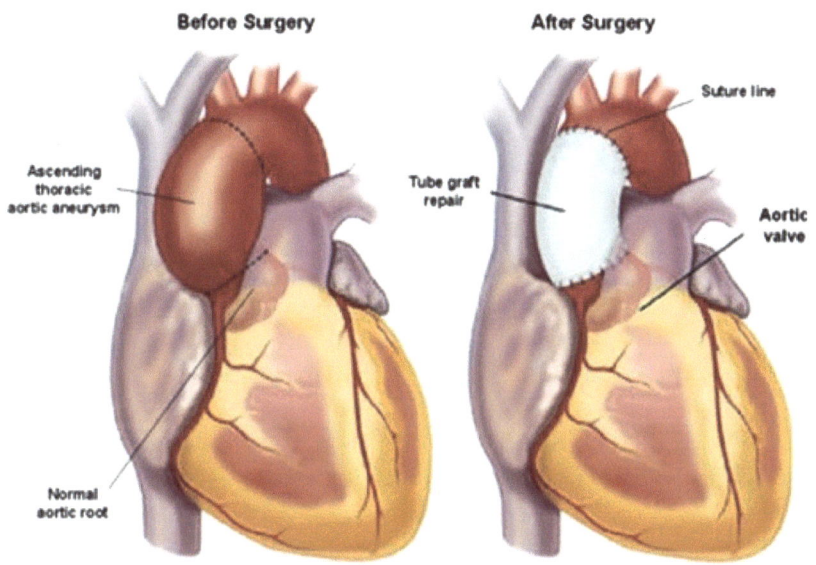

Courtesy of heartguide.com

Table of Contents

Dedication's Page

This book is dedicated to all of the medical

professionals that help their patients with

such diseases as this book discusses.

Brief Introduction

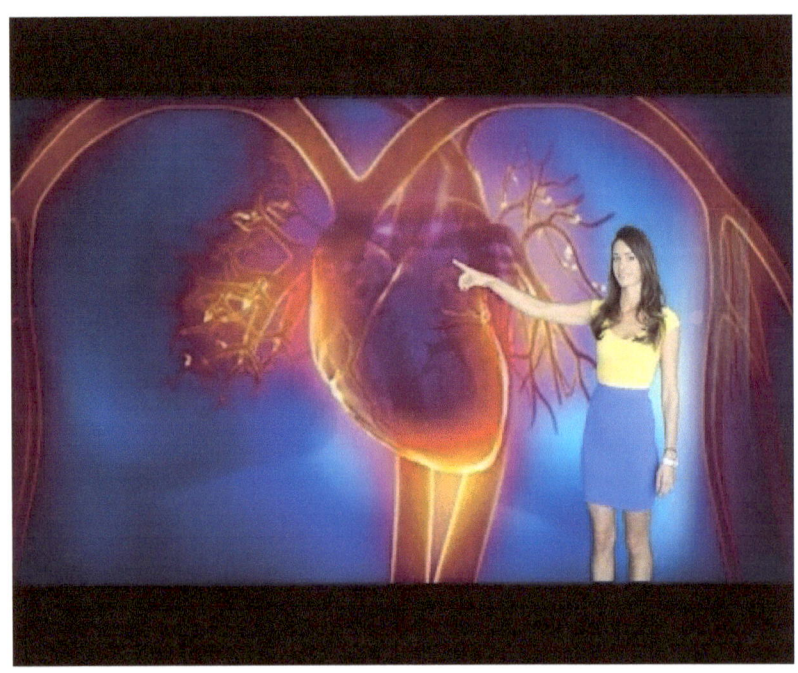

Courtesy of EmpoweRN

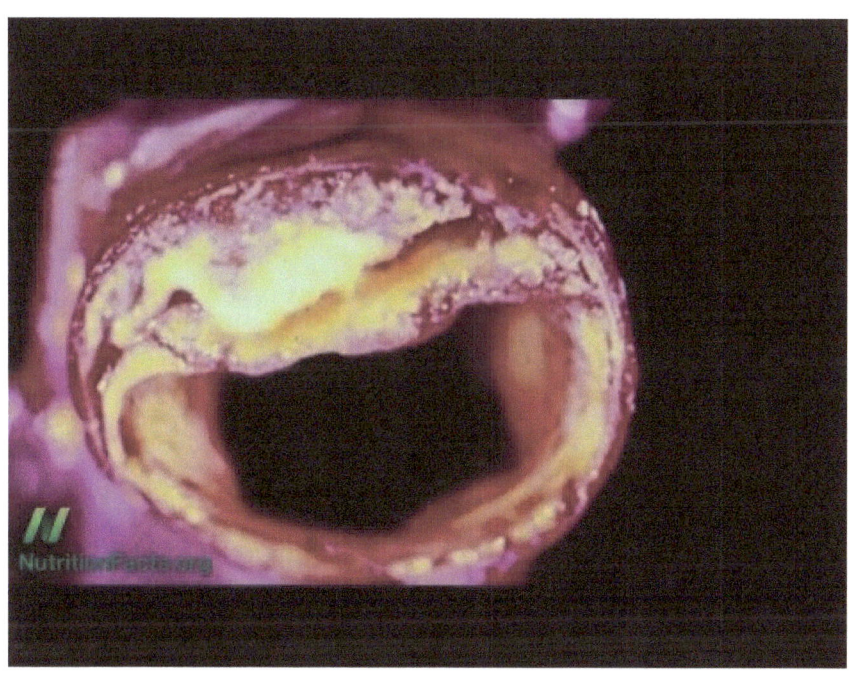

Courtesy of Nutrition.org

An abnormal bulge in an artery of the heart

defines an aortic aneurysm.

Generally, a human heart's arteries are strong

and muscular, which in turn allows them to

withstand a great amount of pressure.

Sometimes, however, an area of weakness may

occur in one of the arteries. This in turn allows

the arteries to become balloon shaped or bulged

in appearance and the artery may push outward.

This is when an aneurysm will occur.

An aneurysm can occur in any blood vessel in the human body but they generally form in the aorta of the human heart.

The aorta is the largest artery in the human body.

Generally, the aorta carries blood away from the human heart and carries the blood to other areas of the human body.

Courtesy of free digital imaging.com

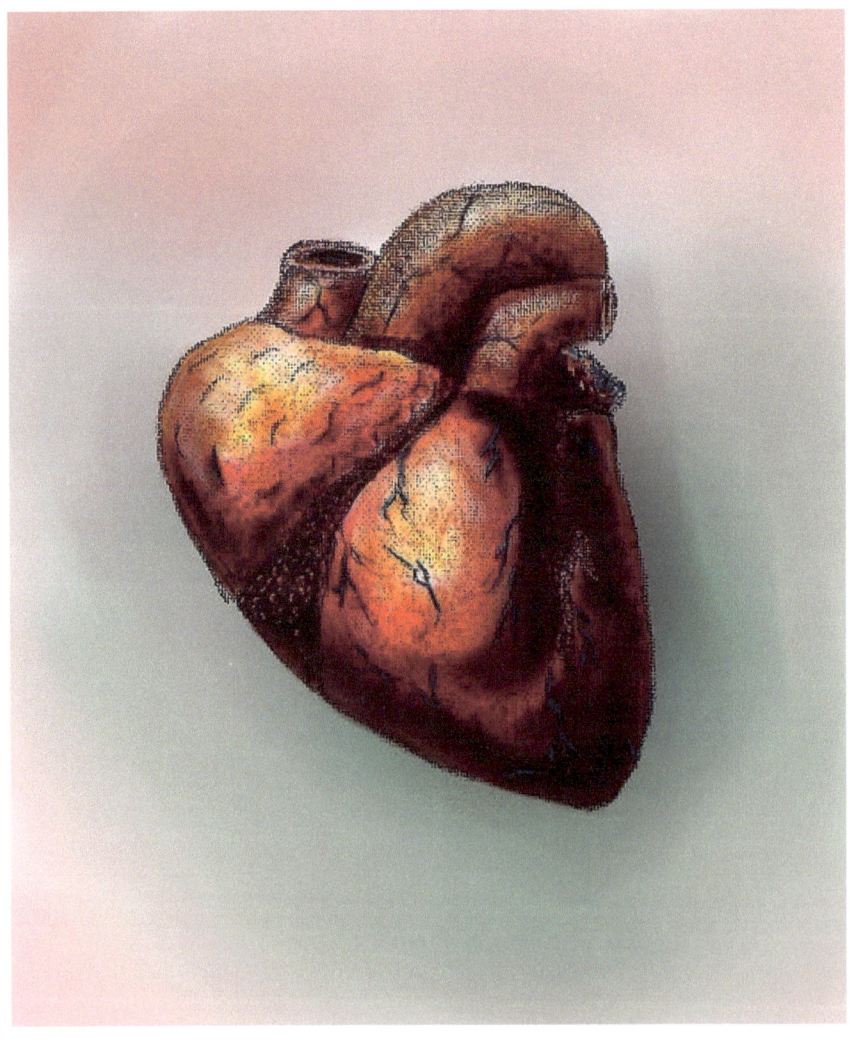

Where do Aortic Aneurysms occur in?

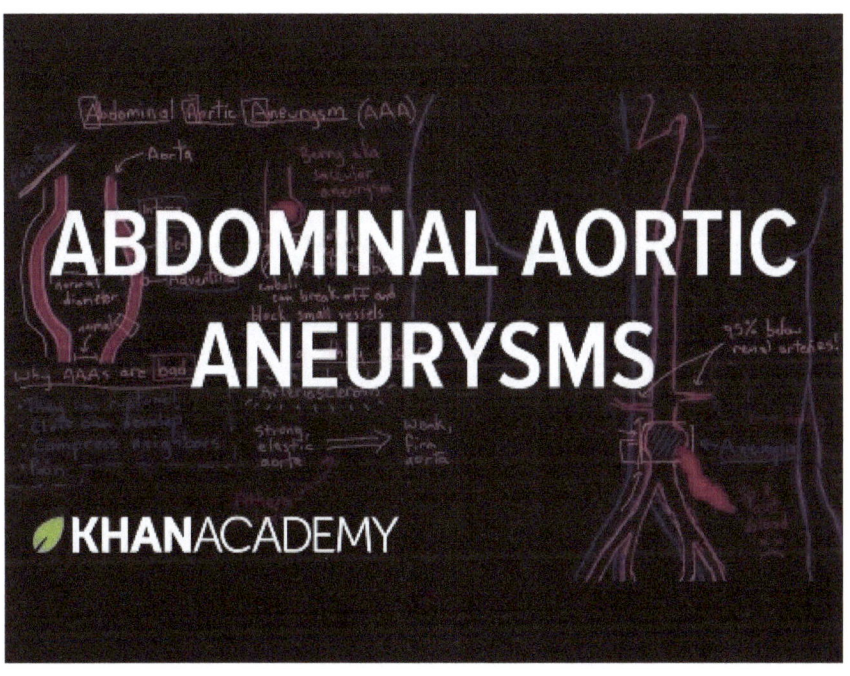

Courtesy of khanacademymedicine

Aortic aneurysms occur generally in two main regions of the human body:

1) Thoracic aortic aneurysms occur in the part of the aorta that passes right through the human chest cavity. These types of aneurysms are less common that the abdominal ones.

2) Abdominal aortic aneurysms occur in the part of the aorta which passes right through the human abdominal cavity.

The abdominal aortic aneurysms generally pass right into the middle to lower abdominal region.

Small aortic aneurysms pose no threat but they can coach along certain risks at times.

Aortic aneurysms can lead to these risks to the

human body

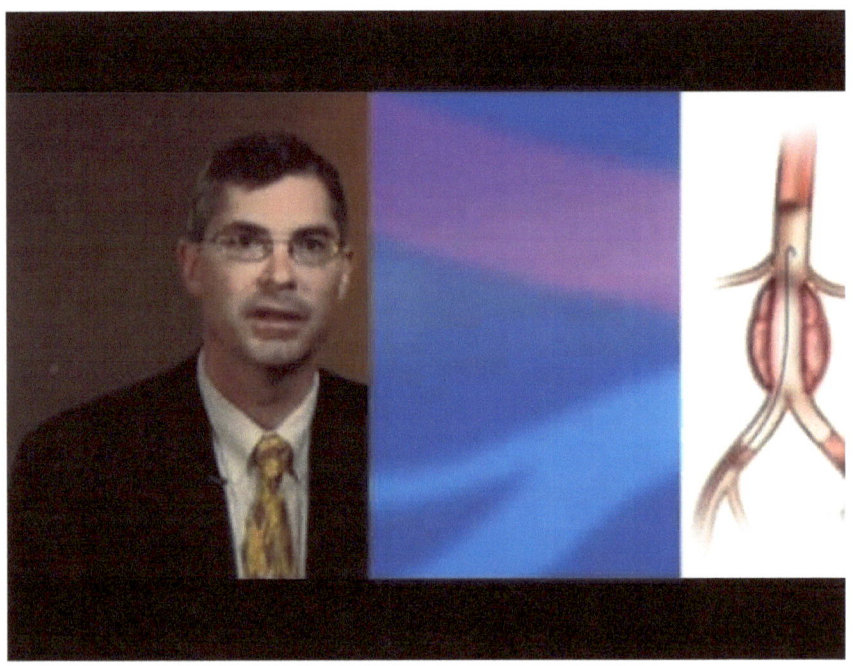

Courtesy of SVS Vascular

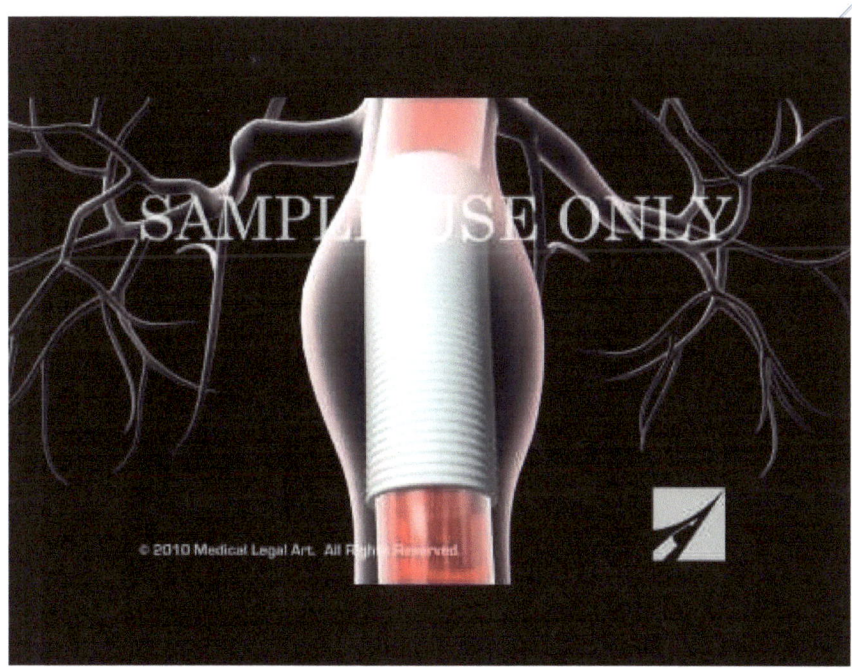

Courtesy of Mayo Clinic

Aortic aneurysms can pose risk such as:

> The aneurysm may move or become dislodged and this can create a blood clot which can cause a person to have a stroke

> An aneurysm could increase in size and push on the other bodily organs, this can cause a lot of pain

> Atherosclerosis plague can form and actually weaken the walls surrounding the arteries of the human heart

> The aortic aneurysm may rupture and this can lead to life-threatening circumstances

Do you know what causes Aortic Aneurysms?

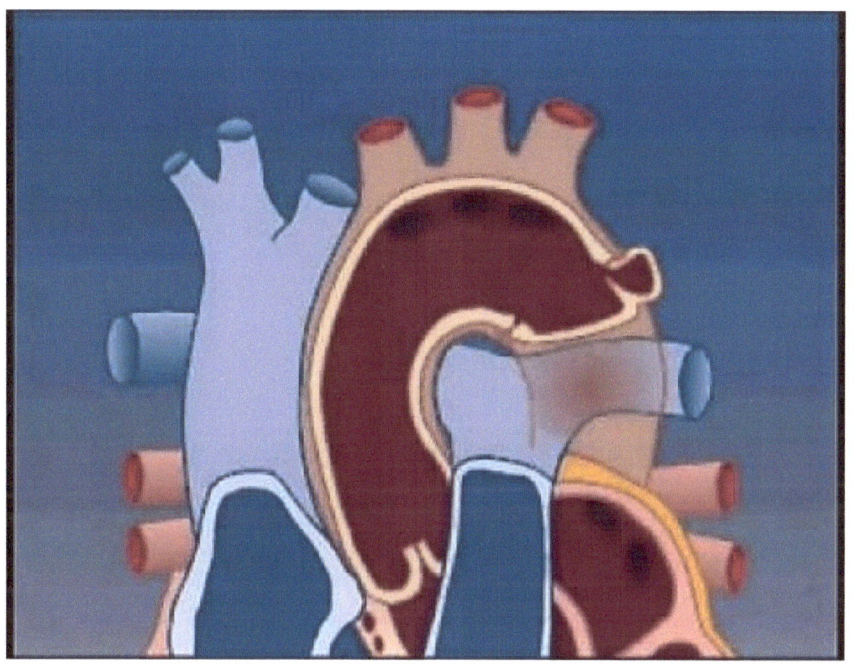

Courtesy of Nationwide Childrens

What may cause an Aortic Aneurysm to form in a

person's body may be:

✓ Congenital abnormalities of some kind

✓ Hardening of the arteries

✓ High blood pressure

✓ An injury to the aorta of some sort

✓ Aging of the aortic artery

✓ Syphilis was also thought to be the cause of

an aortic aneurysm

Do you know if you have any symptoms of an

Aortic Aneurysm?

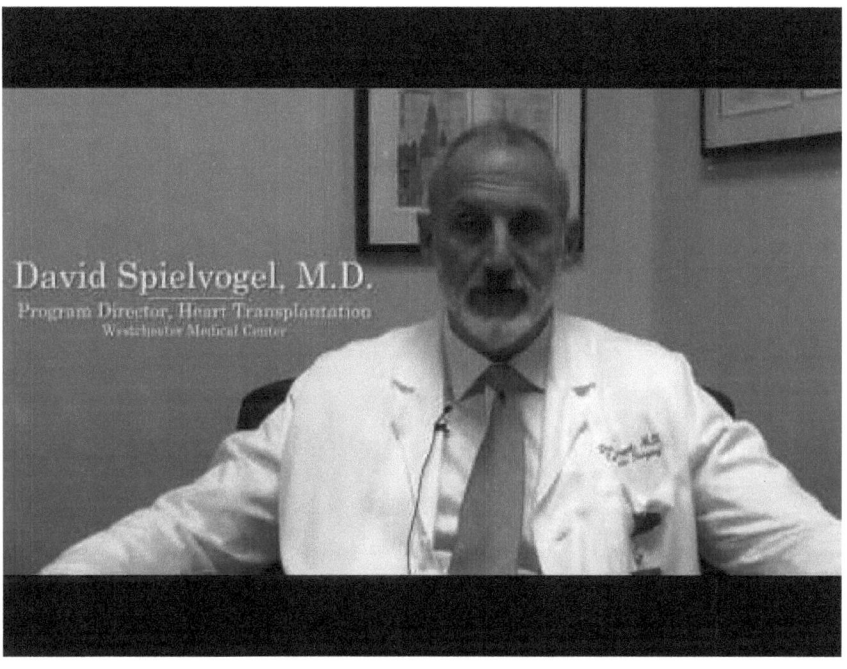

Courtesy of Westchester Medical Center

Some common symptoms of Aortic Aneurysms

may include:

- Shortness of air, hoarseness, difficulty

swallowing, and a cough may be the cause

of a thoracic aneurysm

- Pain between the shoulder blades in the

mid-back region, mid-sternal chest area, or

the abdominal region

- Any rupture to an aneurysm may cause a

heart attack, stroke, shock or loss of

consciousness

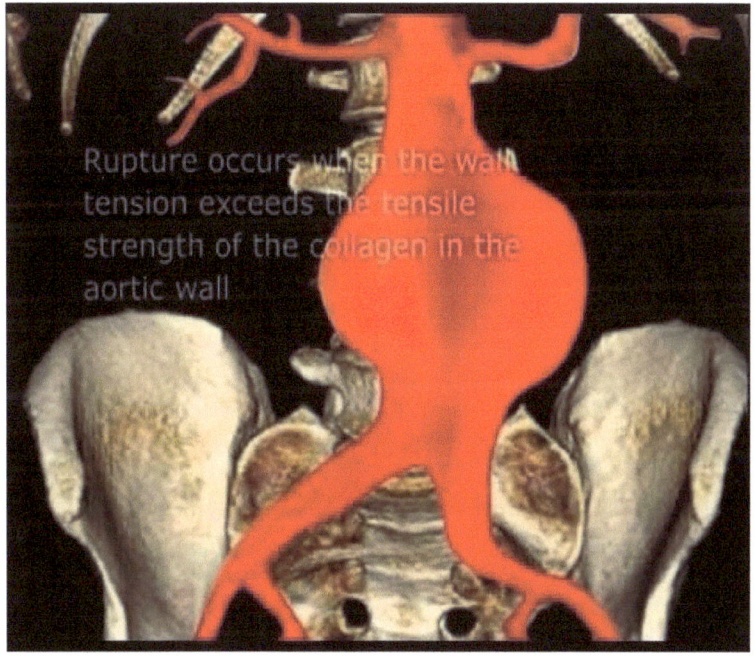

Courtesy of jhcooper02

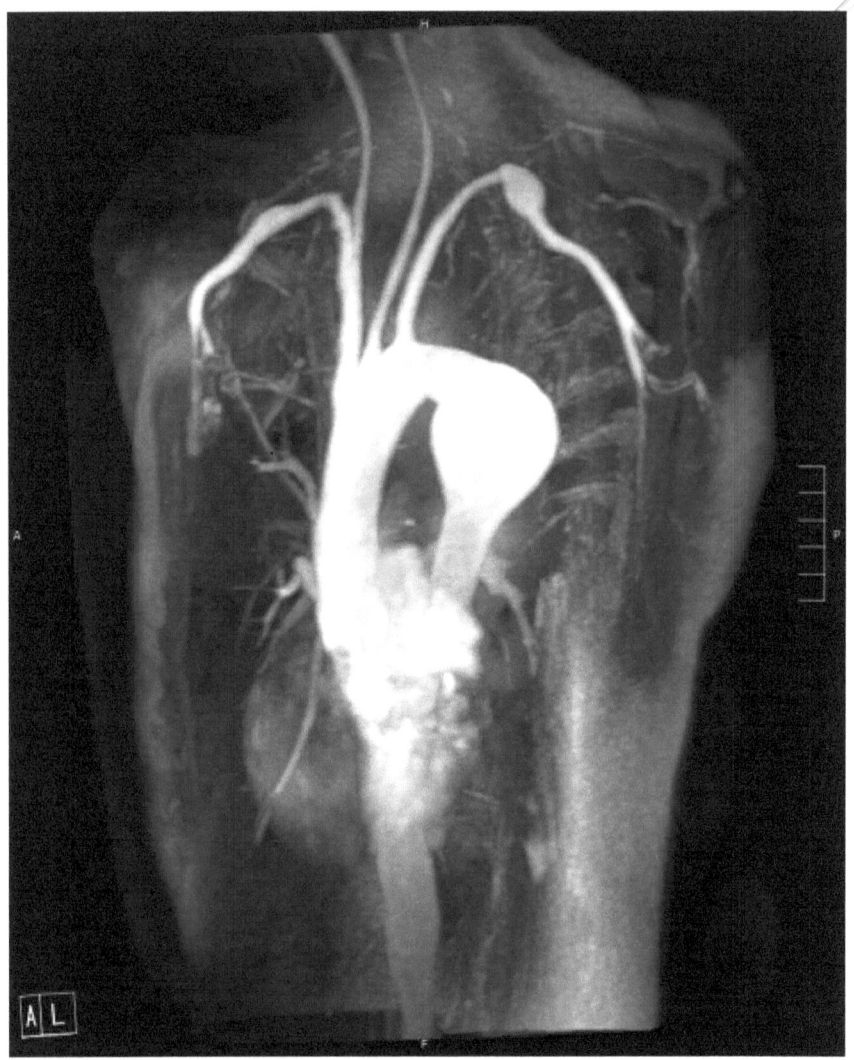

How does your physician generally diagnose an

Aortic Aneurysm?

Retrograde Type A Aortic Dissection After Thoracoabdominal Aneurysm Repair: Early Diagnosis with Intraoperative Transesophageal Echocardiography

Shobana Rajan, MD,* Abraham Sonny, MD,† and Shiva Sale, MD†

Retrograde type A aortic dissection that arises immediately after open replacement of the thoracoabdominal aorta is a rare and potentially lethal complication that has only been reported twice previously. A 74-year-old man with a history of expanding Crawford type I thoracoabdominal aortic aneurysm presented for open surgical repair. The intraoperative course was unremarkable. However, intraoperative transesophageal echocardiography after the repair revealed type A aortic dissection extending up to the sinotubular junction. Subsequently, emergent aortic arch repair was performed under deep hypothermic circulatory arrest. Early diagnosis with transesophageal echocardiography and optimal cerebral protection were instrumental in the successful outcome of this repair. (A&A Case Reports. 2015;4:58–60.)

Iatrogenic type A aortic dissection (TAAD) is a rare but potentially lethal complication of cardiac or aortic surgery. Prompt diagnosis and treatment are essential for a successful outcome. We present a case of iatrogenic retrograde TAAD that occurred after open repair of a thoracoabdominal aneurysm.

Written consent was obtained from the patient for the publication of this case report.

mediastinum. The trachea was intubated with a 41F left-sided double-lumen tube whose correct position was confirmed by auscultation and fiberoptic bronchoscopy. For additional vascular access, a right internal jugular introducer sheath and a right femoral vein central venous catheter were inserted under ultrasonographic guidance. A Swan-Ganz catheter was floated through the right internal jugular sheath to monitor pulmonary artery pressures and to guide

Courtesy of aa2day

Your physician may diagnose an Aortic Aneurysm

by ordering a CT scan, a MRI scan, an Ultrasound

or an Angiogram.

Your physician will watch the Aortic Aneurysm

very carefully. They may recommend that a

repair be done if the Aortic Aneurysm grows over

5 cm (centimeters).

Some Treatments of Aortic Aneurysms

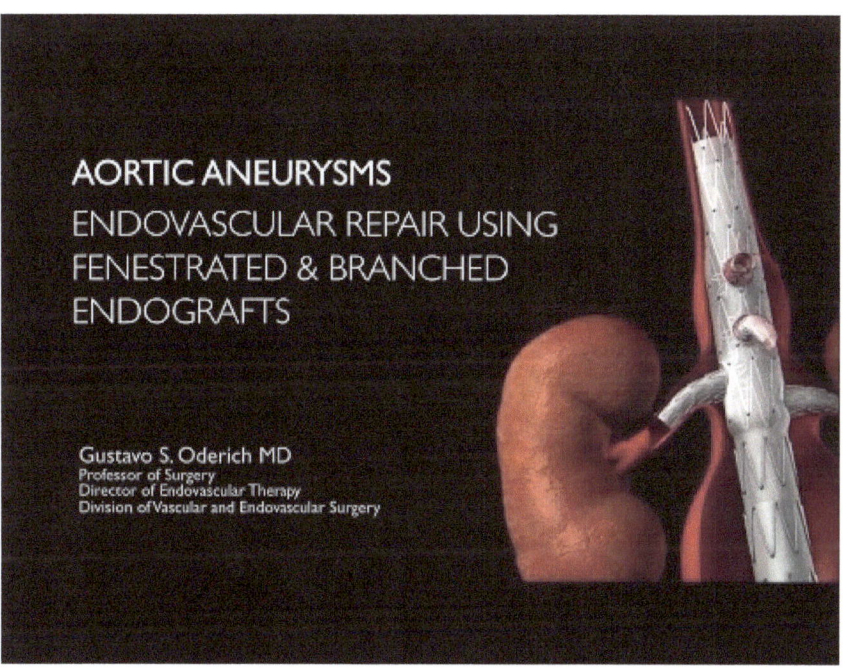

Courtesy of Mayo Clinic

If an Aortic Aneurysm is small, your physician will monitor it closely.

Some Aortic Aneurysms may need to be surgically repaired with a graft of artificial material and if the aneurysm is close to an Aortic Valve, valve replacement may also be necessary.

Newer techniques may involve placing a graft without surgery and a heart-healthy lifestyle as well will be encouraged.

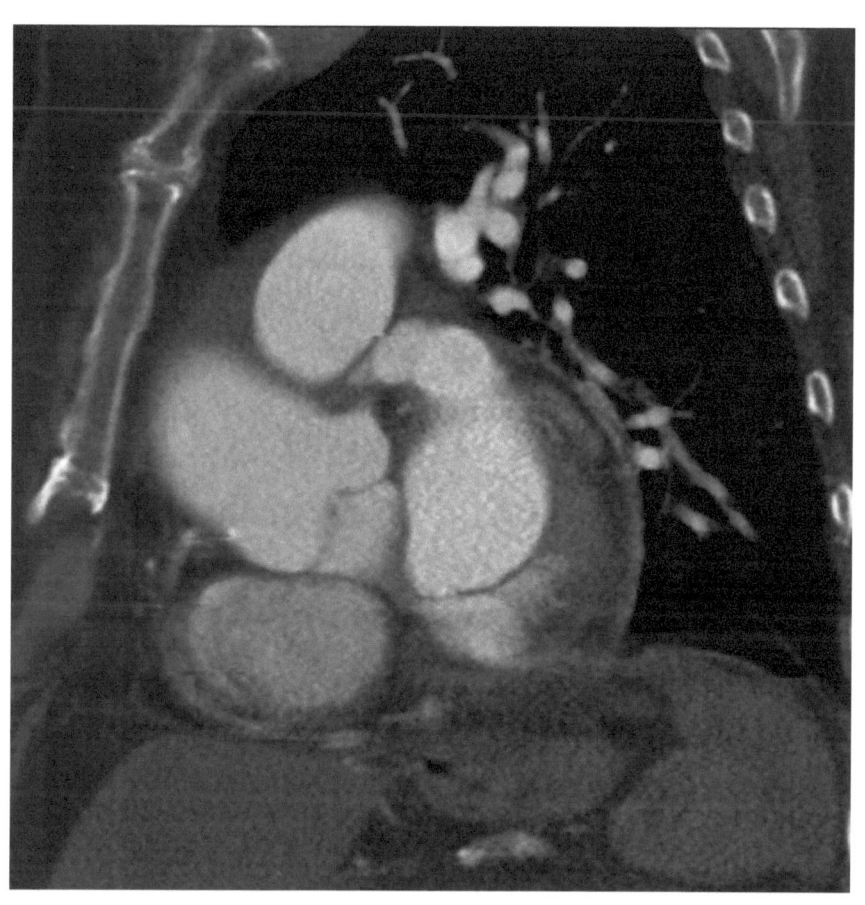

Courtesy of Radiography.org

How to prevent an Aortic Aneurysm from

occurring?

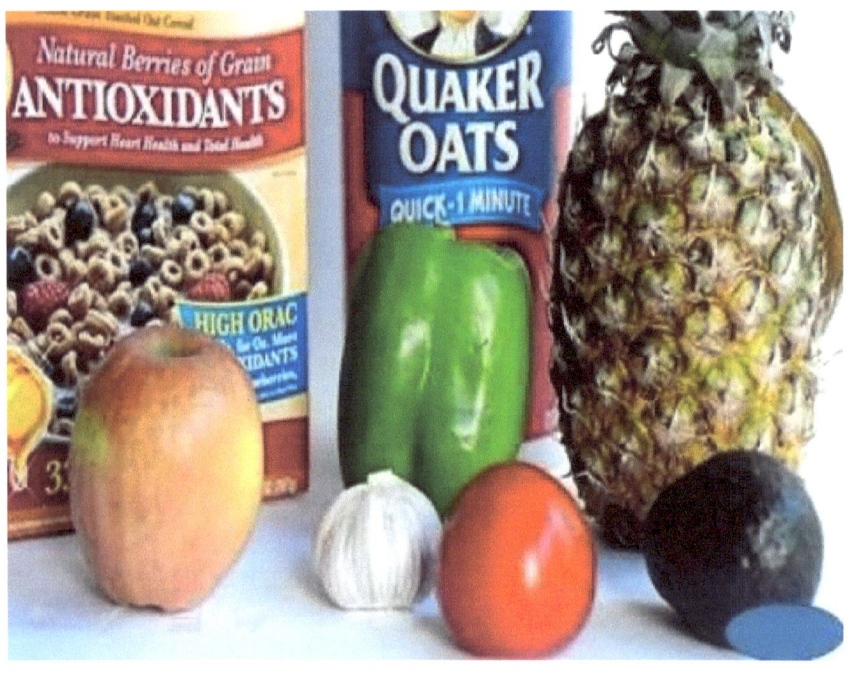

Courtesy of Neshen Jonet

A person can prevent an Aortic Aneurysm by

managing a heart-healthy lifestyle and they need

to see their physician, especially if they have

Coronary Artery Disease or a Carotid Blockage of

some sort.

By following these simple steps, a person may be

able to prevent an Aortic Aneurysm of any kind.

The End

Heart Disease and Aortic Aneurysm is a simple self-help guide to help people understand the disease, how the disease develops, how it is diagnosed and treated and some prevention techniques at a good price. Please take notice that you will have to purchase the online e-book in order to visualize the uploaded videos. God bless!

Misty Lynn Wesley has a diversified career portfolio in the medical, legal, fashion and insurance professions. She is an avid blogger for Examiner.com, Yahoo Voices, and Helium. She also writes articles for CBS Local out of St. Paul, MN and Believe.com sometimes. She has written four books with Publish America and several for

Create Space. The books can be found on Amazon, Barnes and Noble and I Tunes. She and her chosen producers have also produces several audiobooks as well. So check them out if you have the time. God bless!

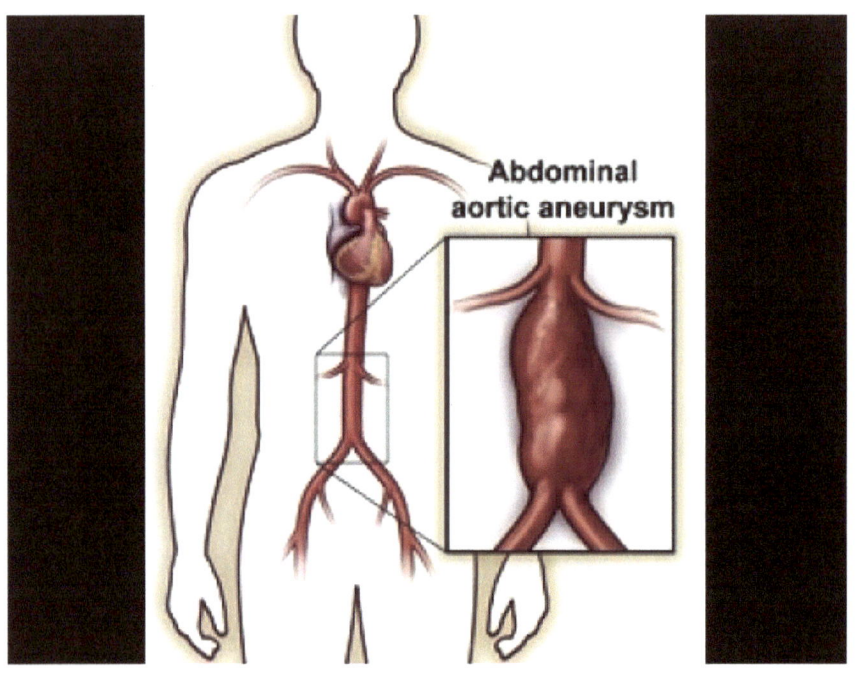

Courtesy of CanadaQBank